the small way

Caitlin Press Inc.
8100 Alderwood Road,
Halfmoon Bay, BC V0N 1Y1
www.caitlin-press.com

Text and cover design by Vici Johnstone
Cover image by Kris Berendsen
Printed in Canada

Caitlin Press Inc. acknowledges financial support from the Government of
Canada and the Canada Council for the Arts, and the Province of British
Columbia through the British Columbia Arts Council and the Book Publisher's
Tax Credit.

 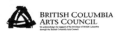

Library and Archives Canada Cataloguing in Publication

Yawnghwe, Onjana, author

    The small way / Onjana Yawnghwe

Poems.

ISBN 978-1-987915-77-8 (softcover)

    I. Title.

PS8647.A78S63 2018   C811'.6   C2018-902198-5

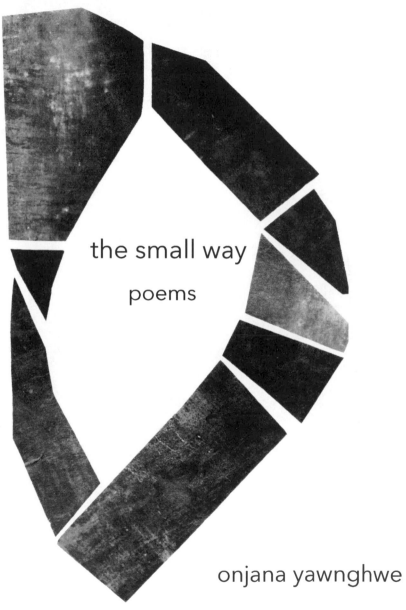

the small way

poems

onjana yawnghwe

CAITLIN PRESS

Contents

Prologue
CHAPBOOK (2004)   8

Poems
ANOTHER COSMOS   12
A QUESTION OF BODIES   13
THE BIG BANG   14
LIMBO   15
THE BEGINNING   16
CATALOGUE   17
HERE TO ANSWER QUESTIONS   18
DEMOLITION   19
PROMISE   20
ROUSSEAU'S TIGERS   21
A STEP BEHIND   23
TIME TRAVEL   24
WE WATCH THE DARK   25
NOW THE WIND SHAKES US   26
CHECK BOXES   27
ALL EARTHLY POSSESSIONS   28
TO BE GRACIOUS IS THE ONLY THING   29
WHAT IF BEGINNINGS   30
OF TIRED BODIES   31
PERFECTION OF SILENCE   32
NOT SUPERFICIAL   34

Theory of Relativity   35
Woman   36
Dead Name   43
Anteroom of Memory   44
Open the Door   45
Selling and Renting   46
Wait for Transformation   47
Coming Out   48
Newest Friends   49
A Troubled Sleep   50
The Elderly Universe   51
Living Together   52
Do Not Think About   53
We Travel Through   54
Skin, Memory   55
Silver Lining   56
Regret   57
And We Kneel Before Heaven   58
A New Universe   59
Waiting   60
Jealous Hands of a Jealous Self   61
We Realize, and Realize Too Late   62
Archeology and the Archeologist   63
Mea Culpa   64
Postcards   65
When I Taught You How to Make Soup   66
Activities of Daily Living   67
The Small Way   68

CROWS THAT CALL IN EARLY MORNING   71

THE MULTIVERSE   72

ROTATION AND ORBIT   74

TRANSPLANT   75

WE MAKE OFFERINGS   76

AS ONCE WE WERE   77

WE HAVE OUR SOUVENIRS   78

NEW LOVE MAKES US   79

THE NEW EXPLORERS   80

HOW TO RECOVER FROM HEARTBREAK   81

NOTHING BUT WAIT   82

ADVICE COLUMN   83

OF PURE AND INFORMED CHANCES   84

THE CINEMATHEQUE   85

WE MOVE AWAY   86

SLOWLY, YOU PACK YOUR SUITCASE   87

RETURN TO SENDER   88

WE PREPARE FOR A LIFE ALONE   89

TAKE THIS RECORD   90

Epilogue

THE PALE BLUE   92

ACKNOWLEDGEMENTS   99

ABOUT THE AUTHOR   100

Prologue

Chapbook (2004)

I

All the retired explorer wanted was a piece of ice to call his home.

This story many people already know; it involves a hurricane, a rich riverboat owner, a pretty girl, and a useless nephew.
In those days no one could accurately predict the weather, so it was not until it started to rain and the river started to heave from the wind that people thought of hurricane.
His plan to break his falsely accused uncle out of jail involved a broken umbrella, a loaf of bread, and a series of hand gestures. Whistling would be involved. But the wind nearly picked him off his feet.

It was said about him that as a child he talked to angels in trees. Because he was artistic, many people expected him to do very many strange things. He indulged them; he loved to make people happy.

She liked to hear stories about him as a little boy, and she liked to hear stories about him as a man. The boy and the man were the same. This is as how it should be, but rarely is.

Under a microscope, lines are rarely straight.

Again and again: we are fooled by what we see.

Sometimes a reader is impelled to be the sole reader of a certain book. So the reader hides the coveted text in an entirely different section of the library: a volume of *Tender Buttons* is placed among books by Julia Child and Jacques Pépin.

The parable of Plato and the cave is retold many times. The tale can be applied to the heart, for example. And he makes up stories. They don't comfort him.

They came to the mountain to climb its peak. But when they arrived, none of the locals could help them. People there thought the idea of climbing a mountain was absurd. A mountain is not something to be climbed; a mountain just is.

A creature just born is unsure of itself. It knows it can experience pain, but also great joy.

II

Her education was impressive, but she chose to forget. Her bare feet taught her the most important things: to step where rain has fallen, to withstand sharpness, to be always ready to dance.

The object of the maze is to get lost and find one's way out through a feat of memory and spatial-navigational skill that scientists insist we are all born with. Many people find pleasure in losing oneself in such a controlled manner. Others panic.

There is always a risk in explanation. Unknown waters birthed sea monsters, dangerous creatures and sometimes even islands. One embarks on a journey with great hope and expectation. Neither success nor failure was assured.

She always believed that she was incapable of staying in one place. Whenever she was on land, the wind and clouds beckoned to her. Yet each place she landed on, she forgot. She imagined what it would be like to be called to the ground, to find some place that wanted her to stay.

In this case, interpretation fails.
Walls are difficult to read, but easy to write on.

Warmth, when it is offered, is sometimes misunderstood.
In glass we see reflections of ourselves.

The girl wanted to play but the boy wanted to dance. But this wasn't a problem because each wanted to give in to the others' desires. But now the girl wanted nothing but to dance, and the boy wanted nothing but to play.

Spring was already on the West Coast. Like a monkey it went from tree to tree. The scent of newborn grass lingered on the necks of women, and even businessmen dreamed in their sleep of sprinting.

Poems

ANOTHER COSMOS

Elements of the periodic table make up four percent of the universe. This is what we know, what we hold concretely, what we build our lives with, in hammer and nail and concrete and lumber. Scientists know little about dark matter, and much less about dark energy, which makes up ninety-six percent of the world beyond earth. We know these things exist because light bends towards and becomes curved.

What exists between two people I know little of. But by the bending of my heart I know a kind of truth. We catch glimpses of another cosmos when we close our eyes. When we finally surrender to sleep, we hold a bright something we cannot see. Was it a singer or a scientist who said we are but stardust?

Inside a person we tread water and wade through bog and craggy morass, encounter women and men huddled under ivy-covered branches. They nod and stare at a small fire, shivering in the wind. You tell the same stories but the narrative changes with every retelling. The way your hands move, the tilt of your head and eyes, the lilt and fall of your voice. The story sprouts a tail, and extra finger, gains spots. You try to tell your story. Tears fall from your eyes.

A QUESTION OF BODIES

Nested within the folds of the self is another self, too shy to emerge.

Within my body, I feel skin sprouting hairs, breasts leaning to the side,
the thickness of belly and thigh, the terrible and debilitating flatness of
my feet.

This is the body I was born and live with,
become an old but indifferent companion.

Your body is not your own.
More a familiar stranger whose kindness you have relied upon but
who, as a companion, has become intolerable.

And yet and yet I cannot imagine the distance between real and
perceived bodies as what a map is to dirt and land.

To put your knees upon the earth,
cheek pressed to the red bark of a cedar tree,
to embrace your wife and feel her chest against yours,
warmth of skins blooming and unfolding.

THE BIG BANG

I thought you'd tell me you were going to die, your face was so serious.
Or you'd fallen in love with another woman, to leave me behind.
These were my greatest fears.
Your face leaked shadows, spilling little light.
When you told me, I felt relief. An ocean crossed my eyes. I thought
you were brave, knowing this dark place you had come from and the
dangerous place you would be travelling to.

I wrapped my arms around you. You wept.
You were afraid I would cut you down and reject you.
But how could I reject the only person I have ever loved?

The land you were standing on was waterlogged and sinking.
You did not know what decisions to make, how you would be in the
world, if you would be transitioning or staying tight with this secret.

I wanted you free. I was impatient for you to decide your life, and thus
mine.
This ache in the background. The world on its head. We were travelling
to the edges of the known universe, where no light would return.
Somehow, our story is ancient.
We were each other's shadow, each taking turns in the moonlight.

There were things to be done.
I swallowed it all with straining mouth, the doubts, the fears, the
unknown, questions of identity, sexuality, stars, satellites, black holes,
supernovas and all the rough cosmic debris.

Limbo

Can we go on as we were?
How can we go on as we were?
I had thought of us as a boring, old married couple that knew
everything about each other. Imagined us as eighty-year-olds: a short
Asian woman leaning against your stooped, tall frame, bearded and
bespectacled. We'd sit at restaurants in silence, attuned to a frequency
that belied words.

It's not as if the future exploded.
It's not as if an earthquake happened and toppled our condo.
No, more like a blankness opened, like someone sliced into time and
tipped open its contents. We couldn't pick up the pieces. A great big
book had been shaken and all the letters fell into a heap.

What would happen to us?
You did not know if you could continue with your face and body.
Your jaw, your chin, your beard, your arms, your strong hands.
Your pants. Your boxers. Your baseball caps.

When a knife is sharp enough you don't quite feel it.
Then there's pain, healing, and scars.
The skin gets so thick that sometimes nerves lose all sensation.

I saw the books on the shelf, read the titles.
Knew the plot and suspected its ending.
And you were still on the floor amidst the jumble of alphabets,
hands scrambling here and there, trying to recover forgotten words.

THE BEGINNING

We make a nest out of
old loose-leaf papers,
cat hair, and dusty books.

I wear your plaid shirt
to smell faintly of you.

We lay on the bed, face to face.
I tell you about my grandfather
who died in a Burmese prison.
Much of my family have gone
unhinged from a grief they deny.
I reveal how difficult it is to live
with this nose, these eyes,
this brown skin, to be always
thought of as foreign.

You tell me about living
estranged from your mother
and sister, how closed up you
became when you were left
with your dad. Kindness was
something you did not experience
as a child. You stopped smiling
at the age of seven.

Both of us have recovered
from anger. We breathe, we open our eyes
no longer turn away from the world.
We breathe. You see me. I see you.
We turn toward each other
toward the world.

Catalogue

Here, a catalogue of my body:
short neck, dark under arms
torso thick, belly soft and jutting
legs that are tree stumps,
finger and toe knuckles hairy.

That is to say I have never questioned my body
like you have questioned yours.

But perhaps question is the wrong word
for the unsettling of a soul.
We all wear our skins differently
but I take this body with indifference
and vague disappointment.

What you exactly feel I cannot know.

Is this what you're going through, a reincarnation?
How to get to the point when the body blesses,
turning instead to the work of decay
and time and the tough work of dying.

Here to Answer Questions

In the beginning you had a need to explain
what 'trans' means, how you know and not know.
You used the metaphor of the jigsaw puzzle,
how you looked back at the pieces only
to suddenly realize that the edges line up
and who you saw in the picture was a woman,
how you were a woman and have always been.

Your father mummified you with violence and
came to you as a ghost inside castle walls,
whispering in your ear poisonous phantoms of yourself,
things that entered your heart and lodged there
for forty years. A new threat for every year.

You lived your childhood with crossed arms and closed fists.
You contained yourself, fastening with locks no one could break.
You thought you'd never grow up to be grown up.
You felt yourself apart from the casual force of men
and turned to the tenderness of women and books.

The self, I don't know what that is.
And how do we know others is another question.
And yet to finally listen to the whisperings somewhere inside.

Here you are, a woman now, grown and young all at once.
How you live your life will be marked on the calendar—
pages turn to newness, entering your new self into time.

DEMOLITION

You say it is a matter of survival,
how you couldn't go on hiding
behind the bearded version of yourself.

I'm frightened for you, I want to cling to you
and never let go. You were assigned to be a little boy.

How you were frightened, how that fear
packed a suitcase and followed you from
house to house, how it arranged our furniture
and barricaded the windows of your heart.

Inside, all the bridges and highways are crumbling.
Nowhere to go but forward and no way to turn back
but to let go. I pick up pieces from the demolition,
mix up new mortar, rebuild. I hand you bricks.

You didn't want to die. You wanted to live.

PROMISE

I told you I could never leave you.
You were the bravest person I knew,
to realize the truth of yourself and your soul.
To realize it and pursue this change,
witnessed before an astonished world.

The effects of estrogen were unpredictable.
You'd said perhaps you would become attracted
to men or feel no sexual desire at all.
But those questions I brushed away.

We do not cry from the promise of a star.
You were my moon and I yours.
We will live together as partners through this.
I want to help you through this dimension,
tend to your wounds and protect you
from the hurt we knew would come.

Rousseau's Tigers

Metaphors are jigsaw
of voices burning, of cats
yowling when all the lights
have been flicked off.

A fist for strength, you gestured,
pointing to the length of your legs.
We were once enrolled in an absurdist school
where Henri Rousseau's tigers grinned
with their clumsy tongued mouths
while the painter waited at the bridge
collecting tolls and writing his long list.

There were pieces that you saw
but you were missing the panorama.
How you felt you always belonged with women.
It can take decades for the world to catch up.

He said it was nature that was his teacher
but he never saw in person the jungles
he would be so famous for painting—
instead we look to what is inside:
the wildness and creatures with glowing eyes
the desperate crouch of winged things
and branches that twist in tropical storms.

Parts of you, I think, spoke:
you a five-year-old clinging to your mother's neck
you so young and separated from your sister
you afraid of what an angry grown man can do
you young and bearded but with tender wrists
you with that engine inside, fiery
you saw the eclipses of yourselves
you turn away I fall behind—

There. Quiet now.
Your head tilts forward in sleep.
In the painting the tiger stoops in fear,
teeth bared, pupils large and stunned
its tail curling upon itself in the gray
and black rain that pummels down,
in the distance brief flashes
string sky to ground, lightning—

A STEP BEHIND

Most people ask why I didn't know,
if there were clues to notice
but it was a secret even you didn't
recognize. Wings flap, crows swoop
at our heads. We held each other
because it was what we needed,
we saw no other selves except for
our own reflections in each other.

But your face has always been delicate
and how I loved your dark, gentle eyes,
the length of your face and your long neck,
the way you held out your wrists,
so nearly feminine and safe for me.
You see, for many years I was afraid of men.

You held me steady in your arms.
You were trembling and afraid when you told me.
Something knocked open inside us.
All I could do was kiss your lips and wrap myself around you
because you did this shaking thing and still were strong.

Yes, I was afraid of this journey.
But in this dark wood
we will walk together.
At first I will be beside you, then behind,
as you take your first steps to live as a woman.

TIME TRAVEL

The night sky is a time machine:
with the knowledge of light speed
we can measure distance and time
from the glimmers of stars.

I think about light and how instantaneous it seems
but when we see the sky we're seeing the past:
the sun as it was 8 minutes and 20 seconds ago
and even the moon we see as 1.3 seconds past.

Personal histories are a kind of constellation.
Patterns of moments that make up a kind of story
as memories coalesce to make a coherent whole.

Like the morning we got married in a Japanese garden
just as the pale cherry blossoms were starting to fall
our small group perched at the edge of a pond
red and orange koi flashing, just beneath the waters.

WE WATCH THE DARK

I need to learn
to relinquish this yearning,
feel you phantom by my side.

All is repetition now,
even death takes on familiarity.

Last night we see a movie
about a young boy in Miami
who lived by silence and
learned to hide, only venturing out
by moonlight to the sound of waves.

You I have worn as armour
for more than twelve years.
You fit me.
Are made for me.

What now this uncomfortable skin,
this yellowness, this fragile sag?

Each of us must meet ourselves in moonlight
determine if there is something to the eyes
touch with inquiry or with kindness,
breaths synchronous as the sea.

Now the Wind Shakes Us

Unsophisticated in the world,
my house had walls and a roof but no windows.
What I thought was sure I was sure of,
matters of men and women and
gender identity and sexual attraction.

When you told me you were transgender
I imagined a window opening, either for
me or you to escape. The wind came in,
shook the pictures on the walls, the cups,
rattled our furniture. I thought of the
wedding portrait my brother painted of us,
two years after our wedding day, each
smiling in each other's embrace among trees.
I thought of freedom and parallel universes.

Could I love a woman? Something in me shook.
I remembered the darkness of my walled house
and shook my head. Was I a lesbian or
something other? Did I somehow sense that
underneath it all, in your eyes and gestures,
your gentle way of knowing, that you were
already a woman? After all, perhaps
that was why I loved you so, for your gentleness
that I could never have found in just a man.

CHECK BOXES

How funny we
   used to think
of boy and girl.

(as if
  not
one thing
   then another)

How absolute we all were—
   as the ink penetrates paper
our convictions fail.

No use in hanging on
   but unclasp and open.

So many ways
  (to think of
   oneself now)

ALL EARTHLY POSSESSIONS

Something in me holds on too tightly:
I've never been drunk
I've never gotten high—
how am I even living?

My own self possesses too much
and cannot abandon with abandon,
and so I question if I ever loved anything
if the person that I loved denies it all.

How we can never forget the performance
of the self, Eliot's *preparing a face* as
the sun breaks down the exhaustion of days.

It's not just gender, it's identity and culture
and the effort of opening our eyes
and continuing on when a darkness pulls
and presses hard on your eyelids.

Once I dreamed you were holding hands with
your future self: a chic well-dressed woman
with a brown bob and black capris.
Beautiful and beautiful.
You were finally happy.

To Be Gracious Is the Only Thing

We are well acquainted with heartbreak.
We surpassed our ten-year wedding anniversary.
You have taken on oceans with your eyes,
textures of sadness you are unable
to name at the gate, waiting to board.

You say it's the estrogen that you're taking
and you are going through another puberty
as if you have arrived in a foreign country
with only a flashlight and a rumpled map.

I am trying to figure out what this shaking
means, this binding of my heart.
Friends ask me, "why aren't you angry?"
but I have swallowed an entire ocean,
salinity and sterile, feelings I can't name
if they are feelings at all.

We take care of the body first
attend to major wounds and bleeds
monitor for concussions and check level
of consciousness every four hours.

WHAT IF BEGINNINGS

I don't know where my husband went
or if I'm allowed to think of "him"—
are my memories of a person or a ghost?
Here and not here, secreting still in my heart.

You say you never think about the past
    (and I don't dare miss *him*).
You are the same person, you say
as if there is continuity between the past and present selves,
like the pages of a book that go from one to the next
and how they form one whole text of a person.

When Italo Calvino wrote *If on a Winter's Night a Traveler*
I wonder if he ever thought about the frustration
of the reader, plunging into a pool
someone quickly pulled the plug from.

I still long to think of you as *husband*:
how steady your arms were around me
how strong and delicate your heart.
We leaned to each other
each swaying like clouds.

These words a eulogy from a faded self.
I am also a stranger to myself as
you are now bright and full of colour,
new and shiny, an explorer ready to embark.

Who am I? Such a tired question
a middle-aged woman should ask.

OF TIRED BODIES

Moonlight runs through our hair.
We belong to our tired bodies
to eyes that close with the weight of time,
we the leftover century, nudging the nibs
and elbows of progress and regress.

You and me.
We defy biological imperatives.
Our breasts will never nurture and feed.
The angles of our pelvis will never ripen.
(I ask myself sometimes if my chosen
childlessness is my failure of womanhood.)

One body becomes another with time.
Hormones send messages to soften
and swell, the skin a soft bed on which
desire is read, written, and become.

PERFECTION OF SILENCE

Over the years, I have perfected silence.
Closed within myself, like a pearl in a shell
that never imagined itself opening to the world.

People glance at my Asian face and place
me in a box, sealed with tape, on a high shelf.
I have become a kind of mistress of silence.
Sometimes I use whips. More often gags.

Except I met you, this person who eased me open
coaxing with words, voice, and careful touch,
until I emerged, blossoming and whispering,
singing Leonard Cohen songs.
To know someone was listening.
To know someone saw through my skin
and name and divined possibility there
was like the moon turning its face
towards other galaxies. Pages open.

You had a psychologist and your trans
support group, and the handful of
work friends and family you'd told.
I was tethered to a particular silence
of the lonely, of the inexplicable.
Dimensions shifted: instead of time
and space, uncertainty and doubt.
Secrets were imposed on me,
it was not my place to tell.
Tears stay close to the skin.
Drop by drop, the sea accumulates.

All the times I made you dance,
swaying myself in your arms,
seeing you unsettled in your body
moving as if a second set of bones
and muscles was controlling you.

You had knit a kind of silence too,
made of guilt and fear of hurt.
The revelation of who you are.

The silence became like ivy,
overgrown and clawed into
bricks and foundations.

Not Superficial

You bring to me the anxieties of womanhood:
is your hair too frizzy, is your lip colour feminine enough,
are these pants too tight, does this sweater look too boyish—
these are things I don't want to think about for myself
let alone for another. So many cracks for women
in this world, worth and value pushed outward.

Who am I to be an example of femininity?

But then I realize these questions are crucial,
part of your survival in this world, these feminine traps.
Dead-end streets and blind corners.
Potential violence in every glance:
your height, your shoulders, your voice

                                        pose a danger—

THEORY OF RELATIVITY

You are preoccupied with the mirror:
how it betrays, how it amplifies dissonance
between assigned gender and gender of the soul.

Your broad shoulders, hairs over your back,
the muscled arms, the thick fingers and hands
with gnarled knuckles, even your smooth voice.

Parts I loved of you,
you wish away.
This is no magician's illusion.
The husband I knew is disappearing.

It hurts to see you hate your body so.
You are eager for transformation,
for hormones to kick in, for curves to show.

What I wish sometimes I cannot say.
Time for you is slow, as the train chugs on.
But to me you are moving
at the speed of light,
blur of blind motion.

WOMAN

1.

We try lipstick colours at Sephora.
I teach you to dab the bullet at the inner skin
of the wrist: crimsons, pinks, and berries.

You're amused by the names of colours:
Amuse Bouche, Desire Me Pink, Arabian Knights.
And textures: glossy, balm, matte, liquid, stain.

Too many consequences in not conforming
to traditional femininity. How to be read
as a woman without surrendering to arbitrary
gender norms, stays, and hooks?
How to express this as your femininity?

—

Hands waver and fingers shake.
You strive to keep steady
as you trace the contours of your lips.

You once told me that as a child
you had won a colouring contest.

2.

The most important thing is to moisturize.
I share with you rich concoctions in glass jars,
white creams smelling of jasmine and grass.
Your skin softens to a milky smoothness
from water and estrogen and skin serums.
You religiously rub sunscreen and stay away
from the sun to prepare for hair removal.
In months you become an immaculate egg,
pale and poreless, looking almost too fragile to touch.

Whether from the skin care regimen,
diet, or hormones, you develop
an inner light that shines from your
body and eyes. Or perhaps it's the happiness
of moving towards who you really are
and who you've always been,
quickly flashing into
the bright sunshine
of womanhood
and being
and be.

3.

The first wig you chose was dark
with blunt bangs similar to mine.
When you wore it we looked a little
like twins, reflected in each other.

I don't think you realized
we had the same hair.
In those early days you wanted
so desperately to be beautiful,
but all you saw was stubble,
wide shoulders, squareness.
Makeup frustrated you.

I wanted so much to fix everything,
to show you how lovely you were,
how your inner self was emerging.
You wanted everything to happen quickly:
hormones, hair removal,
wardrobe, a feminized body.

Sometimes it felt like a train
speeding through the century,
derailing. It was difficult to hang on.
My arms were burning.
Knuckles white.
If I couldn't travel on a seat beside you,
at least I wanted to be on the same train.

4.

In the beginning you wore the skirts
and dresses I kept in the back of my closet
and rarely wore. I was glad to get rid of them.
How strange it was to see the blouses hang on you,
how different my clothes made you look.

From my body to yours.

You'd come home from work,
take off your button-up shirt and trousers.
Dress in long skirts and fitted tops,
your head covered by a kerchief.

We'd go shopping together and began to share
similar taste in clothes. Sometimes we'd even
buy the same shirts, in different colours.
I showed you how a garment flatters the figure,
how with your height you could wear long skirts
and dresses. Salespeople loved you and wanted
too much to help. You were weary of niceness.
You were always remembered at every store.

I think you'd rather not to have been remembered at all.

You have developed an eye for style and fashion
and have surpassed me now. You return with
beautiful, elegant clothes that I could only wear
in my dreams. I'm actually a failure
at femininity, always feeling out of place
among dresses and skirts.

Like a lemon tree
in an orchard of oranges,
longing for sweetness.

5.

You are charmed by your blue Fluevog heels,
kittenish and curved in a vintage pin-up way.

You ask me how to walk in those little heels,
but this is something I cannot help with.

My feet are flat, wide, and ugly,
not made to be squeezed
or compressed by delicate shoes.

You learn to walk for a second time.
You aren't sure if you could pull it off.

As a baby, you were ahead of your age.

Here, you teeter and totter out of frame.

6.

I'm a poor example of womanhood.

We are defined in relation to men, in contrasts:
soft, gentle, subservient, temptress, nag.

Is it the clothes we wear? Our make-up?
Chromosomes mean nothing.

How does a woman.

I know women fight. We are strong
and survive nearly anything.
I know almost every woman has been
sexually harassed, molested or assaulted.
I know in women, innocence gets destroyed.
I know women are used to being
looked at, prodded, judged, desired
ever since they were little girls.

I know women have to pick up all the mess,
gather the loose change, strands of hair
that fall to the floor.

Every one of us puts on a face.

You too have been treated unfairly all your life,
needing to masquerade in a body and persona
not your own. Even other women have attacked you,
in the name of feminism and misogyny. Fuck them.
Cis or trans, we are all vulnerable to the burnt edges
of this strange and violent world. How we are sometimes
killed for occupying these bodies, shades of femininity.
When existing is simply too much.

You have never seen yourself
in portrayals on movies and TV.

There is no correct
way to be a woman.
Only the vague unease perpetuated by
movies and magazines, glossy with lack.

Woman.
She is inside you.

Step into the skin you have always known.
Step into the skin you've always known.
You are a woman, and have always been.

Dead Name

For a period of a few months I don't know what to call you. You have chosen a name, Hazel, from a shortlist we brainstorm together. Vivian, Irene, Ava. Hazel is botanical and somehow suits you. I rehearse the name on my tongue; it comes out hesitantly, with a fade in the beginning and a question mark at the end. The feeling of a borrowed coat. It tastes of sweetened coffee but is lukewarm and strange in my mouth.

A few weeks after you choose your name I buy a mango cake with the inscription: "Happy Birthday Hazel!" You cry from happiness.

Later, you would replace your old name on your birth certificate, licence, all the legal documents. Even our marriage certificate now says I was married to a Hazel in 2006. The paper is crisp and brittle as dried, beached shell. It feels old.

The problem is that I loved your old name, its simplicity and directness, of someone honest, moral, and full of feeling. It's a nice name and hard to give up. Your old name shoots like a star into the sky.

Slowly, you identify with your new name, ask me to use it, along with female pronouns. Slowly, you test out the name in public: at Starbucks, for reservations at restaurants. I see you more and more as a woman emerging from a dark, narrow aging metropolis, map in hand, listening to the strains of music and laughter just a few blocks over.

ANTEROOM OF MEMORY

Is it wrong to remember you as my husband,
so often bearded and shy.
Wrong to remember you as a man
      because you really never were one?

These memories are in some sort of purgatory
    where I sit
perched at the edge of a sofa
      watch for the front door to open.

I wonder

      if I ever knew you

or if I know you still.

Open the Door

The first time you went out
dressed in a skirt and kerchief
on your head I was afraid for you.

It was evening and we walked in
our Burnaby neighbourhood, among
townhouses and low-rise condos.

I was afraid of every look, how strangers
might laugh or make a comment.
I wanted you not to be scarred by this.

But the night was quiet, summer had
settled in and left its curtains open.
A breeze swooped beneath your skirt.

We encountered one man, a shadow really,
who passed us without a glance.
I can still see your eyes, shining in the starlight.

SELLING AND RENTING

After eight years, we decide to sell our condo.
It's not that you felt unsafe
in our neighbourhood.
You wanted to live near other
queer, gay, and trans people,
to become someone more alive.

We rent a two bedroom
on Barclay street and decide
to live together as best friends.
It was hard to see how things would change.

We get rid of hundreds of books.
You donate all your "male" clothes.
I'm too busy to think. I tick off
the to-do list, one by one.

On our way home from the Burnaby mall,
arms full of moving boxes, we see
a man, collapsed on the ground,
his friend yelling for help.

The man's lips were blue,
he was barely breathing.
You called emergency
while I breathed into him
and pushed hard against
his chest, over and over.

WAIT FOR TRANSFORMATION

This paper has no body.
When I write about breasts
they are not mine or yours.

Who are you to yourself?

Who do you see in the mirror?

Who you want to be?

Your skin is as white and soft as the page,
waiting for curves to nudge out in wonder.
You are new and beautiful as a confession.

Yet, time is against you in this puberty
as time is against you and me, this
waiting for mountains to open.

Coming Out

Last year today you announced your transition.
We had settled into our West End apartment,
a bedroom and bathroom for each of us.
We went for a burger at a fine-dining
restaurant, checking reactions on Facebook
and email, both reassured and pleased.

Today, we go for breakfast at 8am.
You get chicken and waffles,
I get a bowl of potato and biscuit hash.
We still live side by side.
We still do everything together.

The day mostly passes as any other.
You say you don't think about the past
and are focused on moving forward.

My mouth is bittersweet.
I don't know what to think about
our love story and whatever is left of it.

Our memories have less and less in common.
Like a 35mm film print in the age of digitization
we see the specks, grains, the imperfections of it
and sometimes the scene flickers to black.

Newest Friends

You make friends,
keep me away from them.
"All we do is talk about sex,
do you want to hear
about trans sex?"

This is new. A privacy
you have built around yourself.
Against me. To keep me out.

I know there is something of
survival to your meeting
with your new friends.
You say you are trying
to build a support network,
one that doesn't include me.

You wear short dresses
and go to queer dances,
pride marches, feminist
book readings. I see
you becoming lighter
and lighter. A strange
weight lifts off you,
your posture straight
instead of stooped.

I feel like an outcast
among the outcasts.
I read. Sleep. Watch TV.
Under an imaginary house
arrest, of which you hold
the lock and key.

A Troubled Sleep

In the streets of yesterday's pride
parade: confetti and stickers and plastic beads.

The beach in the early morning:
    bull kelp, barnacles, and bits of broken shell.

We keep away the lullaby of the ocean.
We keep a troubled sleep.
We think: the sea will always be.
We have our certainties.

Once we were certain we would stay
in our little boat, certain of our quiet life together.
We did not believe we would drown in the waters.

The horizon is somewhere
    we want to go but can never go to.

You'll travel across the Atlantic someday,
fingers entwined with those of your new companion.

THE ELDERLY UNIVERSE

I think it's our wedding anniversary
but we never remember the exact day.

Our status: separated, not divorced.
Living together as best friends.
What does that mean, really?

They say the universe is 13.8 billion years old,
a number we don't understand
in our back-and-forth tattered days.

Subatomic particles arrive
vibrating and disappearing
in and out of our skins.
What does it mean to be inside a person?

Keys jangle in the hallway.
Sometimes the raised voice of an excited child—
sometimes a dog, small for its size, barks.

Living Together

We convince ourselves
that living together will be okay.

      But when you start dating,
living together is not okay.

In fact

      I get jealous
      (don't mean to)

But really, when the girls you date are ten years younger and draw/
write/dance and are delicate and pretty in a totally non-intimidating
way, who can blame me?

I behave terribly. Yell and wail.

      (but am secretly pleased
      to finally feel)

My heart's been in deep freeze
but I'm still alive
la dee la du wop du wop.

Do Not Think About

We were starving for each other.
You were one of the very first people I touched,
how hairs tufted from your body like
celestial nests in a galaxy suddenly near
and how I marvelled at the physics of it all
the long growing length that seemed impossible—

There. A fence around those memories now,
the entirety of your old body, how we touched
and plunged into each other over and over and every day.

I have all these boxes, full of memories of
what I thought was our great love.
They have been piling in our apartment, nowhere to go.
You don't want them, have no use for them beyond
a cursory nod. The past to you now
the pain of who you couldn't be.

We entered into love with pure hearts,
of that I am sure. You were wholly mine
and I wholly yours.
We were naked in each other by the light of day,
lay against each other when the moon rose.
I saw you. You saw me. The moon rose.

We Travel Through

Far from each other now,
I examine the emanations and
radiations of our little love.

We live in the same apartment
but you are years and kilometres away.

In a box I find a tape of the songs
you wrote when you were in your twenties.
I remember them still, the humour and utter
brilliance of them, melodies that somehow
imprint me still. You were as electric
as your guitar, the lights of your mind blinding.

Skin, Memory

How we unzipped ourselves
and collided in the most joyful way.

We watch each other
from either side of the pole now,
your demeanor equatorial,
neither north or south.

The Big Bang happened, there's that.
Worlds pressed and formed
from anguish and wanting.
Explosions and compressions of asteroid
and hydrogen, nitrogen and carbon
are uninhabitable for me.

I limp in and out of orbit around you,
my gait like an aged butler who topples
from too much polishing of silver.

Silver Lining

We fell in love while my father was dying.
Here was a man who was all mind and logic,
books and jokes and slyness,
reduced to a plastic hospital bed with
curtains all around, unable to speak
or tell us the most important things.

I said, *por*, do you know who I am?
Dark eyes stare blankly.
We didn't recognize each other,
each lost in our worlds.

You held me. Kissed me as I cried,
your arms were around me as I dug
into a silence I have yet to come out of.

How tentative your hand
around my waist that first time.

You loving me was the one thing
that kept me from contracting
into a cold black hole.

But now that we have ended
what use is gravity and the rate that tears fall
what use are the kisses and sex and loving madly

and   and

        what use was my father dying?

REGRET

It was my choice
to end our marriage.

Something I couldn't imagine,
being attracted to women.
I saw you as a woman.

Only later did I realize
how you have fused into my heart
how by your mechanism it beats.

I thought it would always be so.
Everything was spinning, you see.
The earth was something to hold on to.

This conventional conception of self was familiar.
It had been hanging there like a dirty
dish towel, flapping in the breeze.
I took it up, raised it as flag.

It was my mistake to think I'd never lose you.
But love and time pick you up and shake
you loose into this new body.
All yours. All alone.
Reaching out. Open arms.

And We Kneel Before Heaven

We become accustomed to the daily rotation of the earth,
pour milk into cereal, recite our daily prayer to get us
up to heaven, the ones that will be saved.

Where does God go when we hear of shootings
or bombs detonated in packed arenas
or when a uniformed hand kills a man
because of the colour of his skin.

We immersed ourselves in such darkness,
see light bend toward it.
It's a struggle to get up every day, a struggle to sleep
a struggle to pull your arms through a clean shirt,
a struggle to put this foot in front of another.

Death may be easier
than this separation
that tears at the stitches
that, so far, hold
this heart together.

A New Universe

Impatient for the decades to catch up, for the world to stop staring
at the genderqueer and trans and intersex and two-spirit and gender
fluid. She imagines this. She raises her fist, she yells. She marches, arms
locked with another, boots stomping in the middle of Burrard Street.
She crosses her arms and gives fuck-you fingers to the police. She
laughs at cis white men in tight dark suits, hurriedly crossing the street
to avoid her.

They would declare, "This is my body" and "Fuck you," and the world
would be wild with it, and start to move, and start to sway in this river
we are all in, this wet current of whateverthefuckthisis, this whole she
and them and you and me and flesh and identity and love and the
whole wantingtobeinsideeachother'sbodies. Yeah.

WAITING

I wait for you to come home from your date
like a defeated general
who didn't know he was in battle.

The chill through the window
reminds me to be reasonable:
let her go

but my heart
plucks me and drops me
in an abandoned city with dilapidated buildings.
Moonlight glances off broken windows.
A cat yowls, over and over, far away.

JEALOUS HANDS OF A JEALOUS SELF

The problem is I want to know, consume every bit of you—
see what you write and who you write to and how you are writing it.
I asked for every detail, every kiss, every fuck,
how you felt the first time you touched, when you knew you loved her,
how your body matched and came together.

Now when I have no claim,
how to live with not knowing,
not be curious with a burning
for the words, the wooing,
the yearning you offer so freely.

A blue hypoxia
on the edges of the mouth.

On the matter of darkness I am an expert.
I desire no one and everyone yet
under my rib cage and between my lungs
my heart still thrums and thrums.

We Realize, and Realize Too Late

I'm curious about your smooth,
creaseless skin, white as bedsheets,
your new breasts. What would it be like
to touch and taste them?
You tell me your body is more sensitive,
even the lightest touch can bring
pleasure, a kiss a gentle explosion.

You have never been more beautiful
than at this moment. A light filters from
your skin, a brightness settles in your eyes.
Perhaps it is a kind of happiness
that I have never seen there.

We both have been lonely,
no one to touch and cradle
and hold us these past two years.
Why have we never turned to each other?

Blame and skin and guilt circle my neck like rope.
I cannot confess it away.
I caused your heart to rip open, while unwittingly
delaying my own operation.

On the steel table, anesthetized,
bathed in the redness of iodine,
skin shaved and draped in blue paper cloth.
Open and bare, it's my turn to hurt.

ARCHEOLOGY AND THE ARCHEOLOGIST

You refuse to speak about
how we were so devoted.
I dredge it up again and again
like a murderous bulldozer exposing
the ancient bed of a river long gone.

Here, I said, was the shape of our sleeping bodies
where we slept entwined, drunk for each other.
Here, the Polaroids that we took of our naked bodies,
the looks in our eyes hopeful and unknowing.

Not having kids made it easier
to disentangle our exhausted limbs.
But little did you anticipate that I wait still,
closed in the red chambers of your heart.

Mea Culpa

The other day you told me about
the mistakes I've made, how right after
you transitioned you didn't like me
introducing you as "formerly so-and-so,"
didn't like how I left traces of your old self
on Facebook. These things made
you uncomfortable at the time but
you were afraid to say so, thinking
you'd put me through enough.

Telling me now makes my heart
fall from its bony pedestal
and shatter open.
What I did was wrong, but only
now do I realize. I hurt
you unknowingly.
For that I am sorry.
I have said sorry to you so many times.

Always trying to catch up,
always leaning against a hurricane.
We were groping blind through
your transition, not knowing what was right,
how much to explain, who to explain it to.

I remove all pictures of you from social media.
Erase your earlier existence from my timeline.
No Chicago, no Indiana nor Amsterdam.
Life from before never existed. Nor I.
The screen is a sterile field.
We scrub the moon clean.

POSTCARDS

We spent our first year on opposite sides of the continent
and every day wrote postcards and spoke on the phone.
For someone who was afraid of men and of opening my heart,
it was a good introduction to love.

Playful, we wrote in code,
inexhaustible and infatuated.
Words leaned and collided with a burning.
Thinking in zigzag, we perfectly understood each other.
We imagined ourselves as explorers of the Arctic,
cataloguing the layers of ice and ancient waters.

And now? And now?
You are ruthless,
never think about the past,
looking only to the future.

On the other hand, I have become an archivist of our love.
Foolish, I know, to remain trapped in glass cases.
But one of us, one of us needs to remember.

WHEN I TAUGHT YOU HOW TO MAKE SOUP

The huge metal pot simmers for hours
filling the air with steam. The apartment
rises with the smell of soup. My family's recipe:
a bean and fish soup from my people, the Shan.

I teach you to boil dried kidney beans,
crush and mince knobs of ginger, roast rice
and pulverize it with mortar and pestle,
stir in a can of tuna, then season to taste:
salt and fish sauce. We make jasmine rice.

We sit next to each other on the blue couch,
large bowls of soup in our laps. Hot spoonful
after spoonful to our lips.
Our throats warm.
Our bellies fill.

Activities of Daily Living

How to make someone want to live?
Is it a mere matter of dopamine and pills?
How to make someone lug their weight
into the shoved morning, dress
and bathe and brush their teeth?

There is no bottom to pain.

If I were all alone I would lie like a stone,
close my eyes and feel the weight
of centuries press on my closed lids.

You were the first person I truly loved.
And the only person I love still.

Neurotransmitters
in this unknown
morse code tap tap tap.

THE SMALL WAY

1.

Once upon a time we dropped
into that Hundertwasser landscape:
its deep green grass, red plots,
and yellow paths that led to the shore
of a river with eye-like flowers.
In our gumboots with pencils in hand,
we followed the steamer ship and greeted
residents with tipped hat and skirted curtsy.

I mailed you a calendar of his paintings,
that strange, tall Austrian who loved the earth.
We looked at images and wrote poems
to each other. The pen was to mind was to heart.
Every day was a reason to wake up.

We were astonished with each other,
your mind nested in the corner of mine.

We walked hand in hand,
fit into each other
as glove to love.

2.

We create a chapbook together,
your poems and mine, back to back.
Dos-à-dos. Back to front. Left and right.
For hours we hand-stitch the pages
together with waxed thread.
We call it "The Small Way."
The index finger separates one page from the other,
but the time between poems is immense.

All around the world,
windows open.

3.

We decide to get identical tattoos
to celebrate and commemorate our love.
The artist adapted Hundertwasser's
painting "The Small Way" in wavy
black lines and tiny squares of blue.

That lost land we abandoned years ago.
Two tattoos, in remembrance.
We vowed to love each other forever even
though our romantic relationship ended.

This spiral on your left inner arm:
do you regret it now?

Does it remind you of too much?

Do you see me in the blue
corner where you left me?

CROWS THAT CALL IN EARLY MORNING

Crows confer just outside our apartment window
with open throats cawing a rawness, bodies shaking.

It hurts to see you so in love with another.
I see the wideness of your smile,
your voice which takes on higher tones.

It is my fault that I have always lived like boxes
taped tight by grief for fear of tipping open.

The clock ticks. I have woken early from a brief sleep.
I hear you sleeping in the other room, your door shut.
We have not shared the same bed for two years now

and yet, and yet sometimes I wish to be held
as you used to do, the whole length of you
pressed against my curled body, the whole of you
the whole of you. The whole of you.

The Multiverse

In this universe you are born
a boy and lived as
a man into middle age.

> In this universe you are born
> a girl and grew into a woman.

In this universe you transitioned
into a woman, listening to all
the little echoes through time.

> In this universe you lived
> obliviously as a cis white male.

In this universe there was no
need to question your gender,
you felt as you were born: female.

> In this universe you are a queer woman,
> seeking the gentleness of women.

In this universe you liked to fuck with
your pants on.

> In this universe you are happily married
> to a woman as wounded as you.

In this universe trans women are
harassed, beaten up and killed
on the street, limping out survival.

> In this universe the heteros are
> at the bottom of the pile.

In this universe people don't stare at you
as you are walking down the fucking sidewalk.

> In this universe men will have tried
> to touch you since you were a child.

In this universe you didn't need to fight.

> In this universe you were born to fight.

In this universe they make survivors.

Rotation and Orbit

How wrong you were when you
said you would be unlovable.

I thought: I will always love you,
at least you will still have me.
We will still orbit each other
in need and want and gravity.

But you have turned and
your turning is fixed.
Your body new and eager to be touched,
to feel and rise to another's hands, kiss
and kiss, devour, blessed in her arms
where it is safe to enter, and good, and
settle, secure and loved and loving.

TRANSPLANT

Replaceable parts:
kidney, cornea, hair
skin, lungs, heart
arms and legs.

I bought you sunflowers after
your father's sudden death.
When I longed so much to hold you.
Your heart was turned toward
another, beating and blossoming
with heat and blood and air.

I used to admire the shine that
quietly set upon your shoulders.
What does it mean to be "just friends"
when you dispense your time to me
like someone forced to go to church
and attend confession, all desire
run out of you, and me secretly
waiting for your love to return.

Love is not replaceable
nor is desire or that burning feeling
that makes you want a person
despite all sorrow and hurt.
I speak now as someone caught
by the edges of a fast river,
scrambling for dirt and rock and
branches among the water moving
towards an unknown horizon.

WE MAKE OFFERINGS

I have tried desperately to show
my tenderest and fragile points.
I clean the house and cook for you,
buy you salts for the bath and wine
to drink. You smile and thank me
mildly, ending with a stranger's face.

And I cannot restore the face that you
fell in love with years ago. I myself
am a kind of dying star, barely visible
with the naked eye, only visible with
a dying eye.

How terrible that I still long for affection
from you who has said, "I can't give
you what you need right now."
Your laughter and jokes and witty bits
of conversation are directed toward another,
where you have landed, as if in a country
where there is no such thing as history
and your memories are but dim and failing
bulbs faint amongst the bright perfumes
of flowers leaning and sighing
to you of the now now now.
And of the past: never never never.

As Once We Were

Your mind was architectural
and wild, always pointing at comets.
Like a magician, you brought me many gifts.

You introduced me to poets I had never
heard of and showed me strange miracles
within the folds of a page.

We have lived together in so many worlds
and walked around the curves of time.
In Thailand, we dodged tuk-tuks and motorcycles
in rough exhaust and nose-to-nose traffic.

What is the distance between here and there?
We read to each other books that we never finished.

I gave you rocks I picked up from the beach.
You brought me to the doorstep of museums,
leading me into colour and perspective and light.

When I showed you the jungle that lived inside,
you opened your arms and embraced it.

We looked to each other, swallowed the words
one another made. We held hands, we touched lips.
The atria and ventricles of our hearts
squeezed and let go, squeezed and let go.

WE HAVE OUR SOUVENIRS

To you I am a foreign place
to which you travelled years ago
but absent-mindedly tucked into the past.

Last year, we talked about writing a book
together, to share and memorialize our love.
But you tire of explaining your origin to strangers
and justifying yourself, as if you were some
immigrant, with suitcase and boxes beneath you.

Now, you are orientated toward Iceland,
hand in hand with your new lover.
In her eyes you see the sea and its horizon.
With her you will explore caves of ice
and glaciers under the Northern Lights,
and make a wish under those green waves
and into the sky for it never to end.

I know: I must learn to let you go
and you cannot force someone to love you.
It astonishes me how well you have cleaved
how deeply and quickly the cut was done.

But here I am, hanging from a hook.
The flesh of my side red, cool, and dry.

New Love Makes Us

When love disappears, where does it go?
Into one of the black holes scientists talk about
where you don't see it disappearing but notice
its absence only by how forks and spoons

lean toward this emptiness.
Our equation is lopsided,
tilted to the left.

Today I buy you a bottle of wine even though
I don't enjoy alcohol, but you have developed
a taste for it, used to drinking with multi-course
meals in fancy restaurants with your new
companion. Hell, you even eat oysters now.

THE NEW EXPLORERS

I can't help but imagine her in your arms
the round softness of her white skin
her full breasts crushed against
your budding nipples, the blond sliding
of her, her pale eyes with irises tunnelling
how your long arms gather and tuck her folds with
the smoothness of your skin and the pelt
of matching rhythm and pace, how your lips
find the tenderness of her and you
press your tongue and hold and hold
and circle and encircle and how her hands
stroke at the heart of you,
around you and inside in between
and how her fingers and yours meet for a second
and hold and cup and hold and kiss with mouths
open, and explore this lovely country
you have found yourselves in, how you admire its
mountains and crevices and rivers and caves
and yourselves, spent, leaning against mounds,
covered with each other's musk
like hungry jubilant animals.

How to Recover from Heartbreak

Today I Google "how to recover from heartbreak."
The first thing is distance, but distance from you
I cannot bear. Being away from you
is like taking a piece of myself
and tearing and tearing into small bits.

I imagine you in every room and tears
drop upon my t-shirt as from a charcoal sky.
I long for the space of you, the infinity of
your stars. You are off to another century,
in a universe of queer women with femme
habits, who hug you and feed you and kiss
you and fuck you and love you as you've
always wanted, deeply and with abandon.

I was seven years old when I came to Canada.
I didn't know I was an immigrant. I found myself
in a land illuminated by a harsh, artificial brightness.
Its creatures laughed loudly and with open mouths.
Some gave me their hatred in little dense balls.
And I swallowed and swallowed, losing every
little bit of myself. I myself am my own cage.

Nothing But Wait

In one dream you are in Mexico
and on the day of your return
you text "Things are so interesting
here. Staying a little while more."

In another we go to a park, but you refuse
to sit on the grass beside me.
You leave abruptly because
she is coming to pick you up
and you don't want her to see me.

Still, I leave the light on for you,
fending off sleep, hoping for a text, a call, an update.
The fact is, we won't be living in the same
place for much longer.
This home we built together,
the furniture, the smells, the air—
you don't want any of it.

ADVICE COLUMN

I haven't seen you in days
but around the apartment
evidence of you. It is difficult
to be among your things,
and the cat here, missing you.

I sit on your bed, trying to conjure you.
The clothes in your closet seem to
wish for a body. The coffee and water cups
in your room: I remove and wash them.

OF PURE AND INFORMED CHANCES

This new love was not what you wanted
or expected. Ol' cupid knocked you over
the head, perhaps causing a small concussion
because your head has been spinning ever since.

That winged creature is cruel
to leave me behind. Directions are
somehow fixed, the wind doesn't
care. The cupped longing of my heart
is none of its concern, nor this sorrow.

I have drunk deeply from the river,
it washes over me in currents.
The heart always declares itself.

You seem so happy it hurts.
You two drink from each other's mouths
never full and constantly wanting.
Her long blond hair curls over you
as you wrap your long arms around hers
and your shoulders hunker in, as her wet
red lips seek your long, soft neck.

THE CINEMATHEQUE

I distract myself at The Cinematheque
watching Éric Rohmer films.
One about a sad, lonely woman
who pushes people away
reminds me too much of myself.
I was a teenager when I first saw his films
and I thought, "Too much talking."
But I realize now how it's not the talking
that matters, but the push and pull of
boys to girls and girls to boys and how
the undertow of longing is the sort of
music that we hear.

A month ago you would
have been at my side, sharing
this bag of buttered popcorn.
What is home to you now,
somewhere with me not in it?

I wanted to see so many things with you:
the Aurora Borealis, Roslyn, Iceland.
I wanted to take you to the Rodin Museum
and show you the tiny sculptures of
Camille Claudel who, unlike her lover,
sculpted what people felt on the inside.

In the Rohmer movies: a tragedy.
One person wants another but
those desires almost never match.

We Move Away

After you fall in love,
my nearness becomes unbearable,
too much skin and prickly heat.

The time has come to live apart.
Our experiment in friendship is ending.
Being in the same room with me
tortures because of my sad face.

I feel I'm losing my best friend.
Within the month we bring up moving
boxes and pack our things
separated and labelled into two piles.

In the final weeks you barely spend
time in our downtown apartment.
I spend my last days with our cat.

After the moves, alone, it takes me
two days to clean the apartment.
I vacuum and mop the dark floors.
Scour the appliances, wipe the cupboards.
Scrub our toilets and tubs, wipe clean
every surface we have ever touched.

SLOWLY, YOU PACK YOUR SUITCASE

When we travel we always leave someone behind. All of a sudden, spring tiptoes in, then summer. Only your new lover makes you forget and feel alive and brings you joy. Not the misery and red-rimmed eyes of your wife waiting for you at home. She tries to keep busy, but that sadness leeches out of her like spilled wine. How it makes your heart twist to come home and see. She makes you cry too often. She reminds you of sadness. You married each other because both of you were broken and you picked up all the shards of porcelain and fit them to make imprecise vessels. You needed each other too much. Perhaps you loved too much. She is in mourning but you are not. Yours was done years ago, when she said she couldn't see herself being with a woman. She was burdened by too much already, it was you who forced her on this journey. No matter. This is inevitable. Now, your passport is ready. You look to the door. You have bought two tickets to a strange land.

Return to Sender

You refuse to take our wedding picture,
the one with you smiling, embracing me
from behind, cherry blossoms in the distance.
Your mother had given it to us, framed.

Today you return the letters I wrote you,
the whole box of them, saying "It will help me move on."
Move from where to where, I wonder?

The day we were married
the sun lit the Japanese pond
and the trees were nearly
exhausted of pink blossoms.
It was April.

We Prepare for a Life Alone

Moving boxes pile up
making a small metropolis
in our small apartment.

We divide up books, paintings, towels,
dishes. You take the coffee maker and crock pot.
I take the rice cooker and blender.

You are barely home these days. There is much to do.
My sadness makes you sad and want to stay away
but you staying away makes me even sadder.
It's unfair of me to show you this hole in my heart,
your fingerprints that linger on my skin even now.

In this city you can walk alone without anyone talking to you.
The sun glints off glass high-rises, making it shine and shine.
I have spent much of the summer in the darkness of movie theatres.

I feel myself growing ugly.
I wish dimensions would open so time
can slip through subatomic particles
and gravity and we could go back.

They say one reality
lives invisibly
next to another.

TAKE THIS RECORD

We had created a paradise for ourselves
but we're human and it all fell apart,
either by design or chance or genetics
we cannot say. We cannot name the cause.

Is it one universe or many more?
Perhaps in some dimension we love,
marry and grow old together until we die.
Perhaps in another dimension we never meet
and pass indifferently as two women on a rainy street.
Useless to try to pierce time and affect physics.

By the rending of the curtain, it is the truth
I desire. I have loved you with every piece of me,
perhaps I do still. We have passed all four corners
of time, have tried to shake its steel foundations.

With these pages, I have entered us into time:
a record that we have loved and existed for
each other for some years. Not catalogue
nor archive. An imperfect rendering from
a flawed and guilty soul. A memorial, an elision.
A dead universe where only the light remains.

Epilogue

THE PALE BLUE

1.

Whatever face and figure you inhabit
whatever desperation that this new life
has brought you, whatever excitement
or fights or hammering of injustices
on your femininity, of showing your true self.

No matter the glares on any random street,
the characteristic swerve of a stranger's head.
To stare, to stare at you. Your body.
You knew the look, what they were thinking.
No matter the everyday indignities of being called
"sir" at a local coffee shop, others insisting on an identity
that isn't there, no matter all that, sometimes
you remember that in a strange way
you are lucky to be able to *be*. To live.
To work and earn money, and walk freely
at day and night amongst those you love.
To hold the small warm hands of a woman
you adore and squeeze tightly to your chest.

2.

I'm sorry that I have to write about you.
I guess I can explain it like this:
we are given the stories we are given.
I don't know how else to understand us,
how we grew and abruptly came apart.

What if our time was all our Sunday mornings?
What you do remember about Leap Day?
I think I want you to understand something
of myself and of how much I loved you.

The recorded messages people sent in
fifty-five languages on the Voyager
were of love and welcome. Enter into me.
We accept you. Come to us.

3.

You will always see me and I will always see you.
Instinct for us to know each other.
You are who you've always been.
The matter of gender that seemed so huge
is really nothing at all when you consider stars.

Deep down we remember the names we called each other,
how it was once painful to spend even one night apart.
We settled into comfort, laid out our rugs.
We work, we come home, we eat. We watch TV.
We talk. We turn on lamps and feed the cat.
We leaned into each other, old skins.

What we don't know makes miracles.
Take lightning and the full, wide moon.
The undulations of the Northern Lights.

We have lived in each other a long time
in the maze of each other's fingerprints.

Being together
was as comfortable
as being alone.

4.

We stand under clouds.
Sometimes rain falls on us, sometimes snow.
Sometimes the wind makes our eyes water.
What will happen to us.

I have loved all of you, no matter your gender.
Because of your gender. I know there is something
within you that will not break. You know.
You will live and make a nest.
You will rest gently and close your eyes.

Remember: your lips upon my skin.
The softness of your side and belly.
Once we held each other with a fury.

We can never be sure of anything now.
Our house is overcome.
All we can do is to leave our hearts ajar.
Do not close. Do not close.

5.

Each other's bodies familiar to us as our own hands.
I know just where to rest my head on your shoulder.
How your fingers can so easily find the hollow of my back.

What to do with all these memories?
Do not imprison them or put them in steel boxes.
It is important to love and remember.
We love because we remember.

Now we bring unfamiliar bodies to our lips.
Now our skins become strange again.

"Nothing can change the fact
that we used to share a bed," wrote D. Berman.
You held your favourite guitar loosely between
your hands and sang to me this song.

We taste unfamiliar bodies.
We hum a familiar tune.

We may be just a blinking star,
dead millions of years ago.
But the light, the light. Still it shines.

ACKNOWLEDGEMENTS

Thank you to Hazel, who gave me permission to include her life experiences in this book. I will always be thankful for the love we shared, and the works we created together.

Thanks to friends and family who listened, talked to me, made me laugh, and who made me feel so loved and valued, especially in the darker moments. So much love to Kris, Sawan, Shannon, Daniela, Ana, Kay, Karen, Everett, Travis, Linda, Darach, Sue, Kelsey, Brigid, and Melissa.

To Betsy Warland, Catherine Owen, and Warren Cariou, who took the time to read the book and provide such thoughtful blurbs: thank you!

Thanks to Vici and her team at Caitlin Press/Dagger Editions. Thanks for your hard work and for believing in this book.

This book is not a transition story. It is the story of a relationship and what it means to love and lose someone. I have only included my personal experiences and my own observations in witnessing and supporting a spouse's transition. I have tried my best to be respectful to the LGBTQ communities in this book and I hope I haven't fallen short.

Canada has so many wonderful trans women writers, including: Kai Cheng Thom, jia qing wilson-yang, Vivek Shraya, Gwen Benaway, and Casey Plett. Their books are beautiful, moving, and make your heart full. Their voices are important and need to be heard.

About the Author

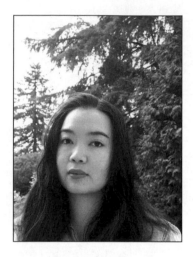

Onjana Yawnghwe is Shan-Canadian and was born in Thailand but grew up in BC. Her first poetry book, *Fragments, Desire* (Oolichan, 2017), was nominated for the Dorothy Livesay Poetry Prize and longlisted for the Gerald Lampert Award in 2018. Onjana has a MA in English Literature from UBC and currently works as a nurse in Vancouver. For more information, visit www.onjana.com.